DIABETES TYPE 2

AND YOU

FIGHT BACK AND WIN

There Is Hope

BY

GREGG PELAGIO

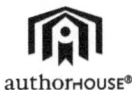

authorHOUSE®

AuthorHouse™
1663 Liberty Drive, Suite 200
Bloomington, IN 47403
www.authorhouse.com
Phone: 1-800-839-8640

This book is a work of non-fiction. Unless otherwise noted, the author and the publisher make no explicit guarantees as to the accuracy of the information contained in this book and in some cases, names of people and places have been altered to protect their privacy.

First published by AuthorHouse 8/14/2008

ISBN: 978-1-4389-0635-5 (sc)

Printed in the United States of America
Bloomington, Indiana

This book is printed on acid-free paper.

This book has been written with my own experiences. These results may not be the same for others. The information is actual and how it pertained to me and how it effected my battle with this disease. Get professional medical help like I did.

Written by an actual Diabetic Gregg Pelagio
and his fight to control the disease

DEDICATION

This book is dedicated to all the people that helped me in my battle to control this disease Type 2.

Dr. Radha J. Mahale and Dr. Timothy H. Martin and the Deer Lakes Medical Staff Oakmont, PA and my Nutritionist, Maryellen Dalmagra Elias, YMCA Natrona Heights, PA.

Thank you!

And to my loving wife Christine who supported me and even went to recommended nutrition school with me and faithfully went with me for months and helped me understand and eat the correct things to survive and combat Type 2.

I Love You!

Thanks,
Your husband, Gregg

TABLE OF CONTENTS

INTRODUCTION

Type 2 Diabetes affects millions of people. It is a deadly disease that if untreated can destroy all your major organs, reduce your life span. So having said that, in December 2004 I was diagnosed with type 2 Diabetes. At 61 years of age I thought the bottom fell out of my life. You will see how I faced it and still staying on top of my regimen. There is hope with Type 2 and You.

Gregg Pelagio

CHAPTER I
WHY ME?

I T WAS DECEMBER OF 2004 I had gotten exceptionally heavy, 350 pounds at 5' 10", but I always worked out. I never thought it was a problem. Well one week I started to get pressure on my bladder and found myself going to the bathroom to urinate very frequently. The fluid was clear. I was having cold sweats and feeling tired. I was always thirsty constantly drinking fluids, water, soda, orange juice, liquids in general. I had a feeling it might be diabetes because as a child I remember seeing a movie where a man developed diabetes in the same way. These symptoms went on for a week until I was feeling run down and made an appointment to see the doctor. When I arrived the anticipation was great. The nurse took my urine sample immediately and found my glucose level way out of control, 485 mg/dl. Not knowing the ranges, I just realized that they said it was high. After I met with the doctor and she reviewed my results she called for blood tests. The blood reveals a 3 month average of your glucose and my reading was over 12, the norm is under 7. So they gave me the bad news I was a Type 2 Diabetic. So with a prescription in hand the staff comforted me and said you can fight it you are strong. They said you are not the first to get it. Why me? I felt depressed, sad, feeling of helplessness. I went home with my wife Christine. She was sad also and hugged me and gave me the support which I needed and said we will fight this together. A lot of things went through my mind. Will I lose a leg, how long can you live with this illness? This is a death sentence. As the night went on I fell asleep. I woke up the next morning thinking it was a dream, but no the sudden reality of the illness was real there sat my prescription of Metforman, a drug used to make up for the insulin malfunction in my body. Going to work was my daily challenge like everyone else. But now I had to start sticking myself with a needle to measure my sugar level. Then guidelines I was given were;

Time of day before meals	Glucose ranges at 110 mg/dl or less
2 hours after meals	At 140 mg/dl or less

These are my targets, your doctor could give you similar ones. For your own goals speak to your doctor.

So here I am I have a needle testing device, medicine to help my insulin shortage and some food comments I was given to use as guidelines and also a recommendation to lose weight. If you are heavy my physician said weight loss would help my insulin efficiency with the medicine they gave me and to continue exercising. Things continued to race through me. God, "Why Me"? I prayed for guidance and help. Well as days went by I was watching TV and flipping through the channels suddenly a show began to air on one of the channels. It was about Type 2 Diabetes. A group of people of all ages were in a room who just had been notified that they had Type #2 Diabetes. They were all hugging and consoling themselves. The biggest thing that hit me was they were crying. As I was laying on the couch feeling sorry for myself a sudden feeling of fortitude went through me and said that's not me, get tough and fight back. So with all feelings of remorse and sorrow for myself I said to myself don't let it take you. This is a death threat so many people do not fight it hard and give up and as time goes by their life begins to fail and before you know it, they have limbs cut off, go blind, have strokes, heart attacks, etc. My wife joined me and saw this program too. I said I am going to fight back and she said I am with you. We can start by finding out more about what to eat. She said I know of a Nutrition school at the YMCA. We can get this information and counseling and fight back. Your right. Now the throngs of Why Me? Why Me? were shelved and the warrior attitude began to surface. God's support was ever prevalent, he showed us the way. Thank you God. My next chapter deals with the battle plan. This was important to surviving and establishing a more quality life. Continue to Chapter II.

CHAPTER II
DEVELOPING
A BATTLE PLAN

I LET MYSELF GET TOO HEAVY. As a child I was always chubby. My mom always had to buy me huskies. When I was about 9 years old my neighbor next door started to weight lift and body build so I got involved in this and thus began my exercise life. I had carved myself out by the time I was a sophomore in High School. Well you know what happens as you grow up you get married, children , jobs, jobs, jobs. Well now in my early sixties with the pressure of the job I put on a lot of weight. I was as high as 350 pounds on a 5'10" frame. Even at this weight I worked out so it never bothered me to be this heavy. But now all of the information I read and my doctor's advice. Weight is a high contributor to Type 2 Diabetes.

So my doctor recommended, understand diabetes and its effects

1. weight loss
2. nutritional eating
3. avoid sugar
4. take your medicine
5. exercise
6. check your blood sugar level daily
7. keep my faith in God

Basically my battle plan, but how was I going to achieve.

<u>Weight Loss</u>

Establish a goal in the beginning I figured I would not set a target/month that was not attainable. Initially set a goal of 1 – 2 pounds each week. How could I achieve this? Well 2 ways came to mind.

A. cut out the calories

B. exercise

Diets as everyone knows are tough so you have to gain the fortitude to become disciplined with your eating habits. My first thought was I will never be able to eat pastry again I loved pastry. My drive to eat pastry was addictive the more sugar and cream the better. I was an actual eating machine. Sometimes 2, 3, 4 donuts at a time. Half of a cake. I really wasn't into candy. So the first thing I drilled into my head was cut out pastry. In my mind I became strengthened by the fact that now I was a diabetic and eating pastry was as bad as eating poison. Pure sugar goes directly to the blood it now stays and is not absorbed by the insulin so this is the situation that starts to attack your blood vessels. It's almost like corroding your pipes (veins) in your body. So that was easy to select so now what. Even diets were no good because they required sugar of some sort so it would not help a diabetic so here I was caught between a rock and a hard place. My wife Christine at this point said they have a nutrition counselor at the YMCA and schooling. So she set up and appointment so we were scheduled to go. So what did I learn to establish my battle plan? Well the first thing os know your enemy. In this case it is <u>Type 2 Diabetes</u>. Weight loss is important. How will it be achieved? Nutrition for diabetics what do I eat that is healthy for me and still loose weight. I take my medicine and check my sugar level at least 3 times a day. So the battle plan in its simplest form was:

<u>Battle Plan</u>

A. understand Type 2 Diabetes

B. lose weight

C. get a nutrition education

D. follow the doctor's orders

E. keep your faith in God and thank him for his support

With all this established it now takes you to chapter III of my experience. What is Type 2 Diabetes?

CHAPTER III
WHAT IS TYPE 2 DIABETES?

My view how it was explained to me and what I read on the internet. Deal with it.

TYPE 2 DIABETES MEANS THAT you have some insulin being produced by the pancreas but the body cannot make use of it like it should. This is worsened by being over weight. Initially the medicine I was given helped me make better use of my existing insulin. Diabetes occurs when you have too much sugar in your blood which can damage your organs. The insulin controls this in the blood. In type 2 you become resistant to the effects of the insulin your body produces. I will not expand on this I am merely telling you what I was told. So the medicine I was given helped improve the insulin I was producing and it helped bring my sugar down. Glucose is another reference to sugar.

<u>Deal With It!</u>

Well now I knew a little about this disease. Now how to deal with it. As I mentioned to you earlier I established a battle plan. Understand Type 2, I am not a doctor or a nurse to simply understand of what Type 2 was enough for me to move forward. So let's cut to the chase. I am following my Doctor's orders take Glucose test establishing where I am. My initial test numbers where high 485 mg/dl, way over the maximums. I didn't even know these limits. All I know was that I was extremely thirsty so I was drinking a lot of fluids water, orange juice, etc. What I found out later is that orange juice turns into sugar rapidly so I was adding fuel to the fire so it actually was bringing my numbers even higher. What a mistake, but how did I know. So the medicine helped to starting to decline it. It does not happen overnight so give it a few days and actually weeks to get it into a normal control level. But all that was in my head that I already worked out. But I let myself go so I was overweight.

Look at my picture on the next page at 350 pounds. Now this leads me to tell you about my weight loss challenge in the next chapter.

Before

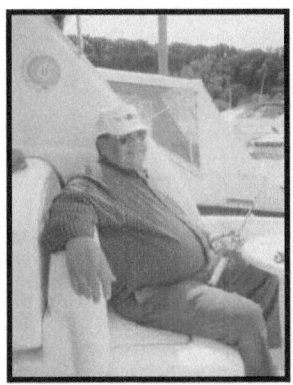

After

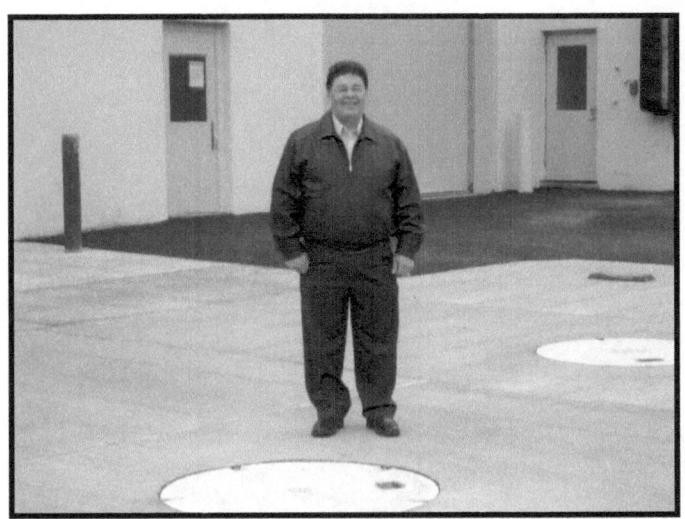

CHAPTER IV
WEIGHT LOSS
CHALLENGE AND
GOOD EATING

Well here I am 350 pounds in body weight and diagnosed with Type 2 Diabetes61 years old and knowing that I want to continue my life. Having worked all my life like all our hardworking peers, I haven't even had the time not to enjoy the life of living without the daily obligation of working. Everyone knows why we work, to get to retirement. No one can predict how long you will live, but God gives us choices and if my choice is to lose weight then if I want to improve my survival in life the "I must lose weight to combat Type 2". It is like my Title Type 2 and You. You like me if you have it must take a strong stand and fight back. Along with my medicine my battle plan was in order fight back lose weight. I am not a laymen of medicine I can only tell you what happen to me, how I Battle this. Again, it may be different for you, but I know my results. In a quick statement so you can get interested I will tell you the results. I lost 80 pounds and reduced my weight from 350 – 270 pounds. My wife Christine had jumped in on the fight and said there is a nutrition course at the YMCA. You can get help there. So she proceeded to get us an appointment. We visited with the nutrition counselor. She was very cordial and said we are here to help you lose weight and eat healthy for a diabetic. She weighed me in at 350 pounds and then we sat down for our first discussion. There is a proper way to eat healthy she said. You must understand what you are eating and the effects of it. First thing we discussed about food was to limit glucose (sugar) content. I did not realize what products turn into sugar faster than others. I was a big pasta, rice, white bread of all types eater. Let me simplify this group. In very simple terms avoid white bread – substitute wheat or multigrain. Do not eat white rice eat brown rice. Pasta avoid altogether.

White or wheat carbohydrate levels are too high. I know you are just as confused as I was so the nutritionist started to simplify carbohydrate counting by understanding carbohydrates you can control your blood glucose levels which will allow you to prevent and reduce the complications of diabetes kidney failure, circulation problems, amputation, stroke, blindness, etc. Yep when you have diabetes we are a walking bomb of destruction and you know what you have to feel that way to be successful. God gave us all a wonderful life and what choices we make can keep it on the wonderful side. Okay let's get back to understanding good eating. For me a diabetic there are good carbs and there are bad carbs. Good carbohydrates for me are those that do not readily absorbed and turn into sugar and bad carbs are food products that absorbed into the blood and readily change into sugar. You need to get a book on carbohydrates and also like I said before take a nutrition course. Again, what I am telling you worked or me. So consult your nutritionist and doctor for their advice.

Bad Carbs (BC) and Good Carbs (GC) for me a diabetic

<u>Avoid</u>

BC – <u>Sugar</u> – products,sugar candy, pastry, or if you eat some look at the label, I use 5g of sugar as a maximum on a label.

GC – I use <u>Sugar Substitute</u> on my cereal.

BC – <u>White products</u> – I did not realize this until studying nutrition white flour, white rice, white pasta, all turn into sugar readily in the blood.

GC – if you desire bread, wheat, multigrain, brown.

GC – brown rice, pasta – avoid altogether brown or white high carbohydrate content. Just to define to me a good carb is made of complex carbs which takes longer to turn into sugar so you end up using this type of carb as energy. I am not a scientist in this field but I know that if this is so I followed it. So to sum it up, for us non laymen scientist eat brown rather than white and your choices for this type of product will help reduce the sugar level in the blood. Starches yield high sugar conversion so what we just previewed makes sense. Rice, pasta, bread and the types we discussed, but also some vegetables produce high sugar corn, potatoes, peas and carrots, avoid when you can. Instead eat salad greens, broccoli, and cauliflower.

Meats and meat substitutes – produce protein. Chicken, fish, turkey, beef, pork, lamb, cheese, eggs, low fat cottage cheese, and peanut butter are in this category. For my own personal choice I eat more turkey, chicken, fish and pork. Peanut butter and carton eggs are cholesterol free. Eat red meat once per week. Now you just don't eat a lot. Everything has portion. So to make it simple as you have heard do not eat more than a piece of meat the size of your palm. Portions – 1 egg, 1 slice of cheese, 1 tablespoon to peanut butter.

<u>Fats</u>

I consume lite margarine if I need a spread. Cook with olive oil because it has been said that it's good for the heart. Also if you need cream cheese, use reduced fat.

Fruits

Some fruits turn into sugar faster than others. This is so involved that you need to study these in a nutrition course. But for me I avoid the following: oranges (which turns into sugar), pineapple, raisins, and tangerines. I eat the following: green apples, bananas, honey dew melons, and cantaloupe.

Beverages

You need to select beverages that are reduced or zero grams of sugar. Here's what I do.

Good	Avoid
Diet soda	Sugar pop
Water (8 glasses a day)	Orange juice
Lite sugar free Cranberry juice	Sugar fruit drinks
Tea with sugar substitute	Presweetened teas
Skim milk	Whole milk
Sugar free decaf coffee	Sugar loaded reg. coffee

All the forgoing information works for me. Consult your nutritionist and doctor for advice.

So without getting into my daily eating plan I want to digress to something very important that I found out. As a Type 2 person I do not make enough insulin to control blood sugar so now I have to do that myself through needle test control, nutritional eating, weight control and exercise. Hey people who think they are fat and have to lose weight without diabetes. If they only knew what we face as heavy Type 2 Diabetics. We have to lose weight as well at the same time control our blood sugar. Now we are in charge of this our automatic systems are gone so now we switch to manual remember check your glucose 3 times a day, once before breakfast, once in the afternoon, and 2 hours after dinner. These are your controls for controlling sugar. Again readings should be:

Under 110 mg/dl before breakfast

Less than 140 mg/dl 2 hours after meals

You will see more of this in the next chapter. These are my limits for keeping a healthy blood sugar level. Check with your doctor to see if he/she has different targets for you. But I was told these are the guidelines. Now what I was digressing to well here it is you must eat at least 6 times a day, 3 snacks and 3 meals and here's why. When you are controlling you sugar sometimes we drive it too low and this is called low blood sugar. When it gets too low say under 70 mg/dl for me, I get cold sweats, start to shake, blurred vision, and if it gets too low I want to pass out. Having the snacks keeps me on a more controlled level. This whole eating thing is so important. You have to take a nutrition course as I said to understand it.

So here is what I was given for me to lose weight. Control my sugar and become healthy. Remember once you get Type 2 it will never be cured, but you can fight back and prolong your life. We all have choices in life. If it is too survive then buckle down and start a positive attitude. My menu and what I do to lose weight and control my sugar. First of all throw out the word diet. This is a life style change. First of all my calorie intake was set at 1800 calories per day for my size. Smaller people will have lower targets. The next thing was to understand carbohydrate counting. The most important thing for me as a diabetic is balance carbs with protein. A carbohydrate is equal to 15 grams so if someone says eat 2 carbs = 30 grams and 4 carbs = 60 grams.

Breakfast

4 carbs or 60 grams of carbohydrates

So I have to weigh my food. Once you understand carbs you will be able to judge, but in the beginning weigh your food in grams so you can get the correct grams of carbohydrates. Remember carbs give you energy and the right carbs keep you healthy and your blood glucose in control now you also can read the labels. When I went to nutrition school we spent 2 ½ hours just reading labels. You will see on a label grams of sugar, grams of fat, grams of carbohydrates, calories, etc. Again when you see on the label 15 grams of carbohydrates his is referred to 1 carb. Now you need a blend of starch, fruit, grains, etc.

So for me breakfast is simple.

½ cup Bran Flakes – 1 carb

1 banana – 1 carb

1 cup skim milk – 1 carb

and I use a ½ teaspoon of a sugar substitute. So for breakfast I have consumed approximately 50 grams of carbs.

10 AM Snack

Protein – choices:

1 slice of cheese

1 egg

3 oz of cooked chicken, beef, or pork

¼ cup of cottage cheese

Lunch

Again 60 grams of carbohydrates

2 slices of lite wheat bread – 2 carbs (remember no white bread)

1 green apple – 1 carb

1 teaspoon of lite margarine = 5 g fat on your bread

You are allowed 3 servings per day of fat 5 grams per serving.

2 oz. of meat again chicken, pork, beef, tuna, etc. and lettuce, tomato – 1 carb

So basically I have a lite wheat bread sandwich with 2 oz. chicken, lettuce, tomato with a teaspoon of lite margarine spread on the bread. Now for a beverage I have a diet soda or water. Remember no sugar drinks just look at the amount of sugar and carbs on the label. Sugar is a no! no!

Snack 3 PM

1 oz. meat or meat substitute

Look back at the choices

3 oz. cooked chicken, beef, pork, turkey, or fish

1 egg

1 slice of low fat cheese

Dinner

60 grams of carbs

3 oz. of meat

non starch vegetables

5 grams of fat – for example:

     1 cup of honeydew melon – 1 carb

     ½ baked potato – 2 carbs

     ½ cup of cooked vegetables non starch – 1/3 carb

     1 glass of skim milk – 1 carb

Total 65 grams of carbohydrates

Last snack – 7 PM – no later

6 Ritz low fat water crackers

plenty of water

Everyone knows this one, 8 – 8oz. glasses of water today. So now you see what I eat for a day. Again, I am not an expert, but you must gain some knowledge of what you are supposed to eat. Again go to nutrition school to learn about these food groups.

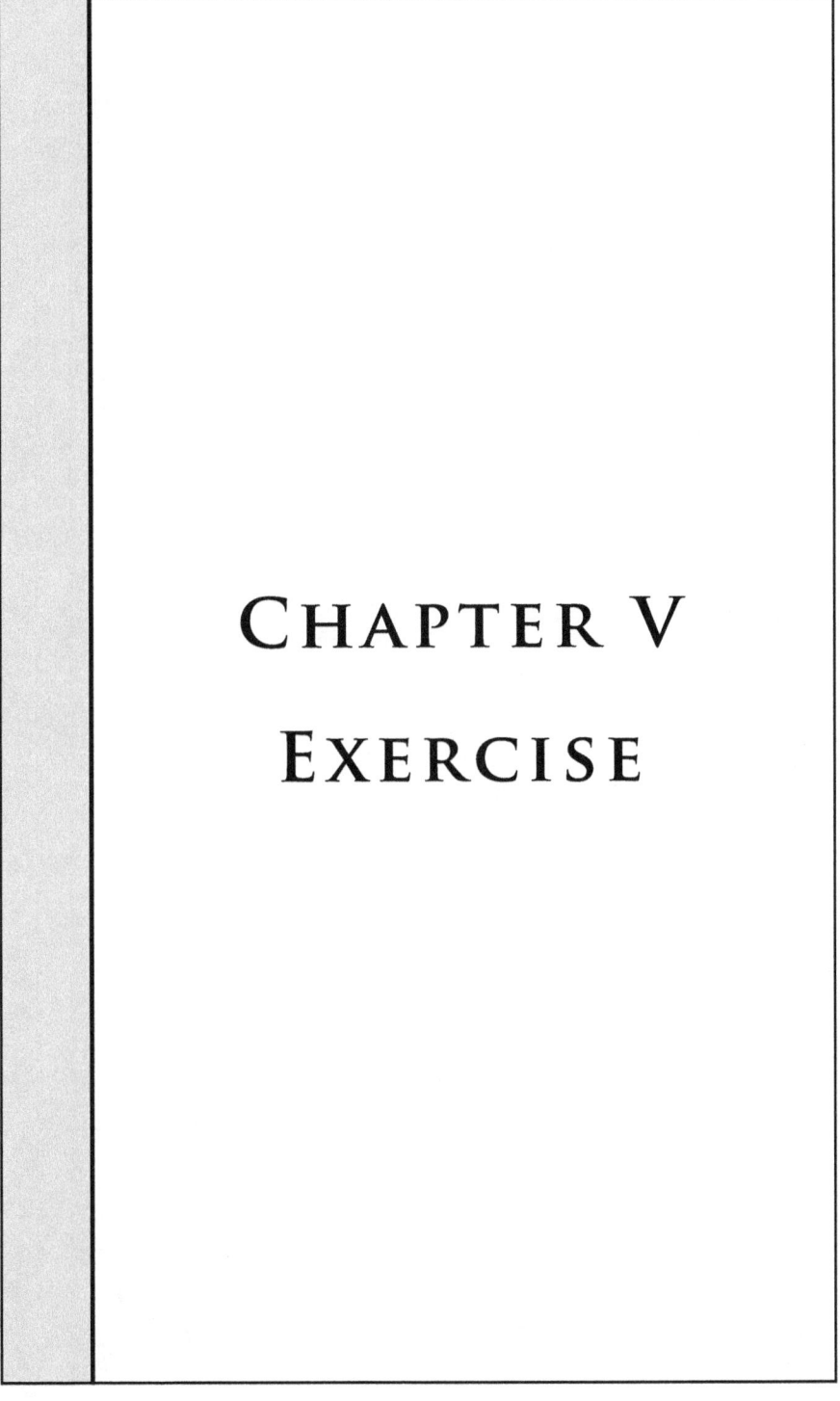

CHAPTER V

EXERCISE

CONSULT WITH YOUR DOCTOR TO see if you are healthy enough to workout. As part of my life I always exercised. Well having been a regimented gym guy when I was in school the usual things happened to me growing school, job, family, etc. Well now I worked out even though I was 350 pounds, but as you can see I was not very well built. And as you know I became a candidate for Type 2 Diabetes. Physicians tell us to help yourself with Type 2 lose weight and it helps considerably. Working out also tones your muscles. You know we lose muscle mass as we age. So keeping muscle tone and maintaining this condition is good for your health and vital organs. So here is what I do again ask your doctor first if you can involve yourself in exercise before you begin. I am a morning person I do my workout before I go to work which I am normally in my office by 6 AM so my workout starts at 3:45 AM and is completed in about 35 minutes. First of all there is the cardio workout for me get he body warmed up get the heart beat up and get the blood circulating through your body. I purchased a low impact cross country ski machine. There is a foot to foot shuffling and hand an arm motion similar to a cross country skier. There is no impact so your eyes are safe. You know how they say you can damage your eyes with hard ground contact of the feet pounding. Well I don't worry here so I do 10 minutes at a brisk pace on the machine. This gets my heart rate up and I feel everything loosening up and getting energy. After this I keep a fast pace going. I have a sit down sit up stomach machine which I briskly use for another 5 minutes. After this I take a 2 minute break and do some controlled breathing. I take breaths through my nose and exhale through my mouth. This helps get my blood pressure down so I can prepare for my weight lifting workout. Weight lifting is what I do. You could buy one of those gym systems, etc. My weight lifting consists of 3 sets of light weight squats 100 – 135 pounds to the lowest point minimum 10 – 12 reps/set. 4 sets of bench press weight that I am comfortable with, 4 sets of 10 repetitions. 3 sets of standing presses. 10 reps each of: 3 sets of bicep curls and 3 sets of reverse curls. Your workout depends on what you want to do. But some form of resistance exercise is good for muscle tone. I do my repetitions slow because I was told it should help my HDL cholesterol. Exercise in general I have been told helps control my diabetes.

Chapter VI

Measure

Your

Blood Sugar

M Y TESTING DEVICE IS MY life controlling unit for keeping my blood sugar out of the danger zone. All devices come with a record book, record your readings date, time, and reading. Let's show the guidelines that I follow from my meter. They say they are published by the American College of Endocrinology. So matching what my doctor told me, these are my guidelines.

- At 110 mg/dl or less – Before meals
- At 140 mg/dl or less – 2 hours after meals

Glycemic A1C Control Limits (3 month average)

Glycemic Control Limits

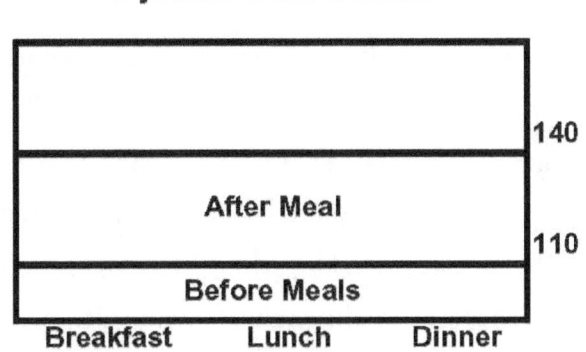

These targets A1C are consistent with the goals published by The American College of Endocrinology consensus statement on guidelines for glycerin control Endoc Pract. 2002 8 (Suppl 1) 5-11 check with your doctor for your own guidelines.

---

*These values are suggested by the published guidelines of the American College of Endocrinology.

*Check with your own doctor or healthcare professional on what target range is best for you.

My doctor requires a fasting blood test every 3 months which test my for my 3 month (A1C) average of sugar (AACE* recommends under 6.5 A1C).

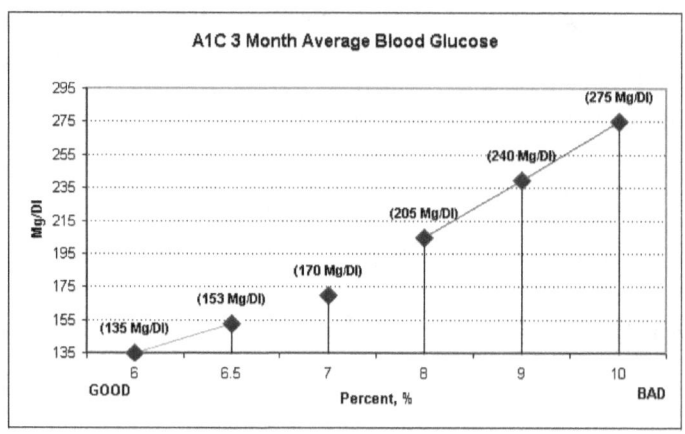

So reading your blood is like checking the oil in your car. Too much is not good, but there is a safe level. So I test my sugar level when I get up before I eat breakfast. I try to stay between 95 – 105 mg/dl. This is my personal target. Before lunch under 110 mg/dl, 2 hours after any meal less than 140 mg/dl, right now if you are a new diabetic your readings in the beginning are higher. The readings you see me at are after the medicine and weight control kicked in with the exercise. You must get a relationship between what you eat and your readings. Make sure you record what you ate and keep a record of all your test readings.

---

*American Association of Clinical Endocrinologists relationship between average blood glucose and A1C.

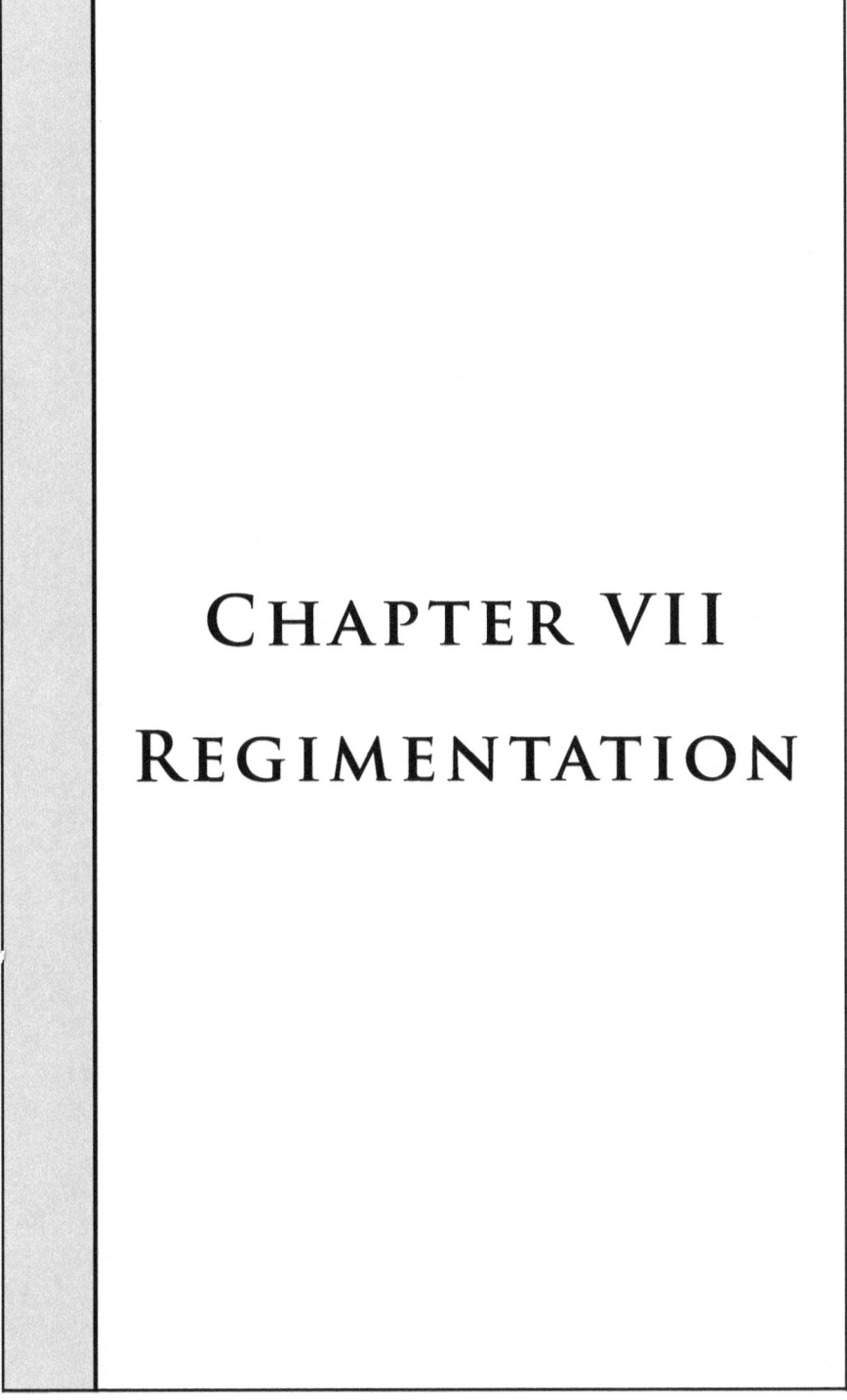

CHAPTER VII
REGIMENTATION

So now I have the tools to deal with my diabetes. This is a new way of life for me. I must regiment my life style to where food is necessary and life is more important. What I am saying as a heavy food connoisseur I loved to eat a pound of pasta with a lot of meatballs. I was a pastry eater. More, more, sugar pop or soda as it is called, white bread, Italian French bread, white rice, pasta. No! No! No! It was all about taste. Now you have to create a mind set so you can go on with your life. I had to set a regimentation that I had to accept and now I live this life.

<u>Regimentation</u>

1. Weight control – I bought a scale. I weigh myself daily. I set a limit of +5 pounds when I hit that I reduce calorie intake.

2. I test my blood 3 times a day to make sure it is not getting out of control. At the 3 month doctor visit a blood sample is taken and my 3 month average of A1C is tested. When this number is available my doctor let's me know. If my number is under 7 I am in control, 6 is nominal.

3. Every 4 months I go to the foot doctor to check my feet for color, good circulation. As a Diabetic your feet will show initially if circulation is being deprived. Your nails will change color, your feet will loose sensitivity. So a sensitivity test is done to see if you can sense the feel.

4. Every 6 months I get to the Ophthalmologist (eye surgeon). He reads my eyes to see if the sugar is attacking my vision. A series of tests are done.

5. Periodically a kidney test is done to measure the effectiveness of your kidney function.

6. I exercise 5 days a week, Monday – Friday, with the weekends off.

7. I renew my understanding of nutrition by reading books and going to visit my Nutritionist with follow up courses. I attend seminars. I talk to other Diabetics, we share information. I try to encourage them as well.

8. I maintain my faith in God whom has supported me throughout this Diabetic disease challenge. Keep a strong partnership with him and you will survive. Hope, hope, hope. With all this you may say well is it worth it. Look around life is beautiful. We are lucky to have a second chance at it. You, like me, need to choose to do the correct things. With this it brings me to my final chapter, what happened to me. Again, this is what I do. Check with your doctor for his/her recommendations. This may not work for you.

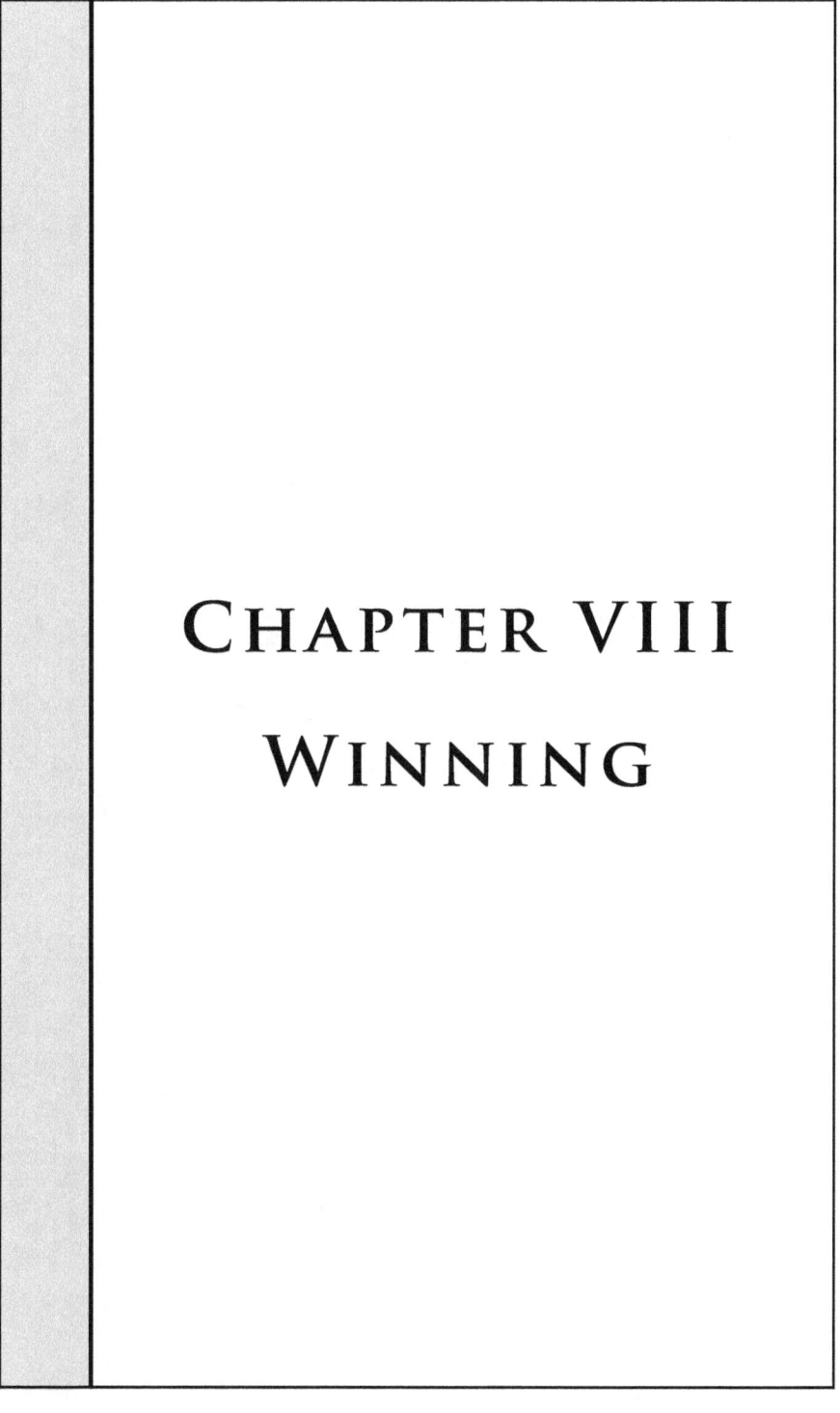

CHAPTER VIII

WINNING

WINNING THE BATTLE OF TYPE 2 Diabetes is and always will be a challenge for me and anyone with Type 2 Diabetes. I have such a story to tell I even tell my wife I would love to be on the Oprah Winfrey/Ellen DeGeneres/Rachael Ray show or a TV network show to tell a wide audience that there is hope. You must not get discouraged. That you too can beat back the carnage of this disease and keep it in check. You can, like me love your life better. Enjoy the daily things of eating for health, exercising, and making the correct choices. For this was my results. After 1 year because of my regimentation I was able to eliminate the use of the Type 2 Diabetes medication, for a year and a half now and I am controlling my sugar level with:

- smart eating habits 6 times a day
- exercising 5 days a week
- keeping my weight in control after losing 80 pounds
- checking with my doctors regularly
- thanking God for his support

I hope you found my story positive and makes you want to take care of your yourself like me. Only you can reach out and fight back this tough disease.

God bless you,

Gregg Pelagio

About the Author

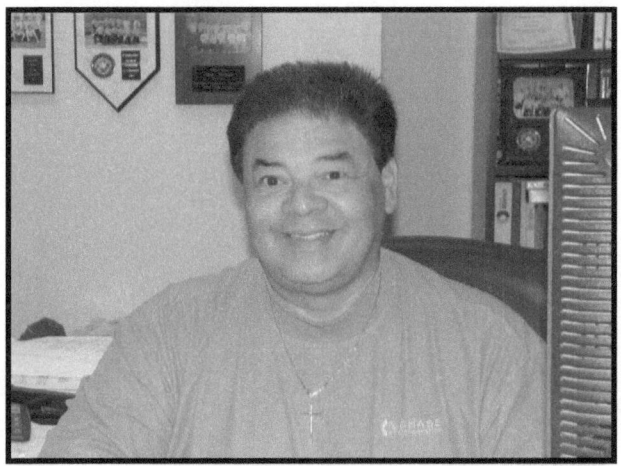

I GREGORY A. PELAGIO AM YOUR everyday American who is not a celebrity or any paid actor. I am like you and everyone who faces the daily challenges of life. I am a family man with a loving wife, 3 children and grandchildren. My position is a working manager and provide for my family like everyone else. Type 2 Diabetes was my health challenge. There are so many unsuspecting people that will develop this disease, maybe reading my book will help you prevent getting Type 2 Diabetes. Those that have Type 2 Diabetes hopefully reading my book will help you control yours. <u>Diabetes Type 2 and You, Fight Back and Win.</u>

"God Bless You All".

Gregg A. Pelagio